A Year in Color

	J	F	M	A	M	J	J	A	S	O	N	D
1												
2												
3												
4												
5												
6												
7												
8												
9												
10												
11												
12												
13												
14												
15												
16												
17												
18												
19												
20												
21												
22												
23												
24												
25												
26												
27												
28												
29												
30												
31												

- ☐ IRRITATED, FRUSTRATED, OR ANGRY
- ☐ NERVOUS, STRESSED OR ANXIOUS
- ☐ ENERGIZED OR EXCITED
- ☐ CALM OR RELAXED
- ☐ DEPRESSED, SAD OR EMOTIONAL
- ☐ ACTIVE, FOCUSED OR MOTIVATED
- ☐ HAPPY, POSITIVE OR OPTIMISTIC
- ☐ TIRED, RESTLESS OR UNEASY

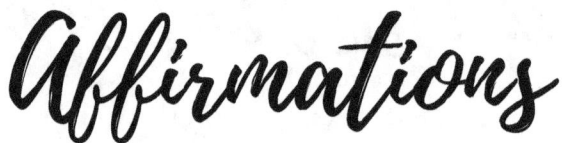

DAILY AFFIRMATIONS

IDEAS & PROMPTS

I'm in charge of how I feel today, and I'm choosing to be happy.

I'm brave enough to climb any mountain.

I have the power to change my story.

I've decided that I'm good enough.

No one can make me feel inferior.

My strength is greater than my struggle.

I'll use my failures as a stepping stone.

It's not their job to like me. It's mine.

Success will be my driving force.

The only person who can defeat me, is me.

I dare to be different.

I do not need other people to be happy.

I deserve love, happiness and success.

I am loved and I am wanted.

I will not apologize for being myself.

Positive Thinking

POSITIVE THOUGHTS:
WRITE DOWN YOUR FAVORITE INSPIRATIONAL PHRASE

Do what makes you Happy

AFFIRMATION:

One Day at a Time

JANUARY

S	M	T	W	T	F	S
		1	2	3	4	5
6	7	8	9	10	11	12
13	14	15	16	17	18	19
20	21	22	23	24	25	26
27	28	29	30	31		

NOTES & REMINDERS

One Day at a Time

MONDAY'S MOOD

TUESDAY'S MOOD

WEDNESDAY'S MOOD

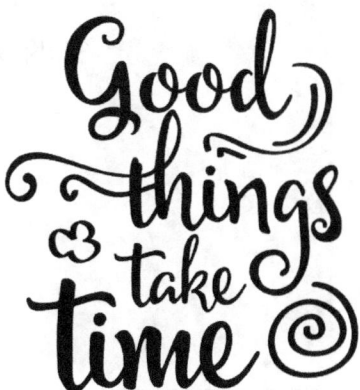

THURSDAY'S MOOD

One Day at a Time

FRIDAY'S MOOD

SATURDAY'S MOOD

SUNDAY'S MOOD

THOUGHTS & REFLECTIONS ABOUT THE PAST WEEK

My Mood Today

DRAWING THAT DESCRIBES YOUR **FEELINGS**

It's just a bad day, Not a bad life

Positive Thinking

SELF CARE TO DO LIST:

- [ ] _____
- [ ] _____
- [ ] _____
- [ ] _____
- [ ] _____
- [ ] _____
- [ ] _____
- [ ] _____
- [ ] _____
- [ ] _____
- [ ] _____
- [ ] _____
- [ ] _____
- [ ] _____
- [ ] _____

PHYSICAL NEEDS

EMOTIONAL NEEDS

HOW I FEEL TODAY

I WANT TO WORK ON...

Self Care Checklist

GOALS M T W T F S S

Got enough rest

Spent time outdoors

Drank enough water

Spent time doing Something that makes me happy.

Went for a walk or exercised.

Spent time with family

Meditated

Connected with friends

_____

_____

_____

NOTES:

Mood Meter

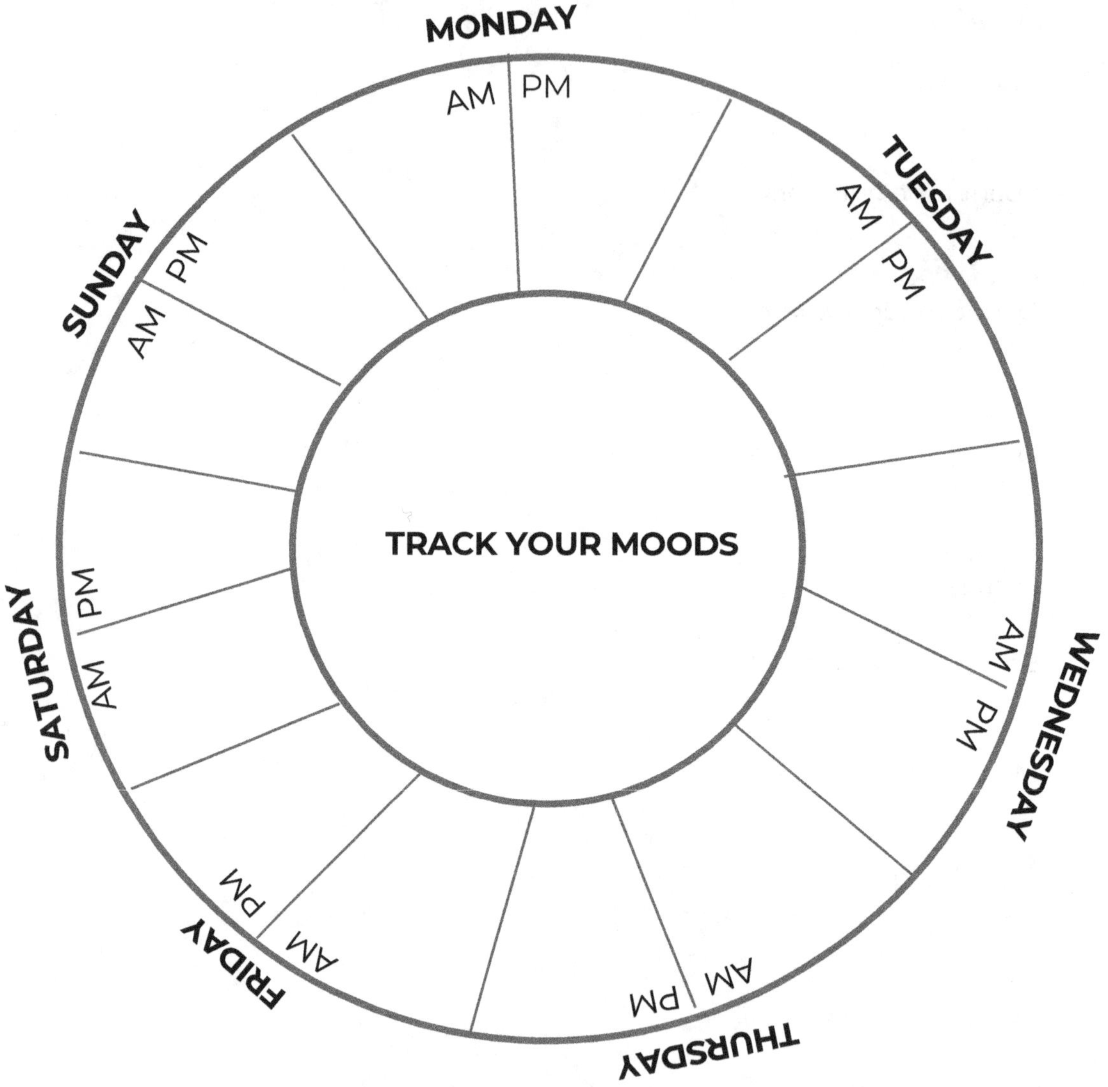

MONDAY — AM | PM
TUESDAY — AM | PM
WEDNESDAY — AM | PM
THURSDAY — AM | PM
FRIDAY — AM | PM
SATURDAY — AM | PM
SUNDAY — AM | PM

TRACK YOUR MOODS

COLOR SCALE

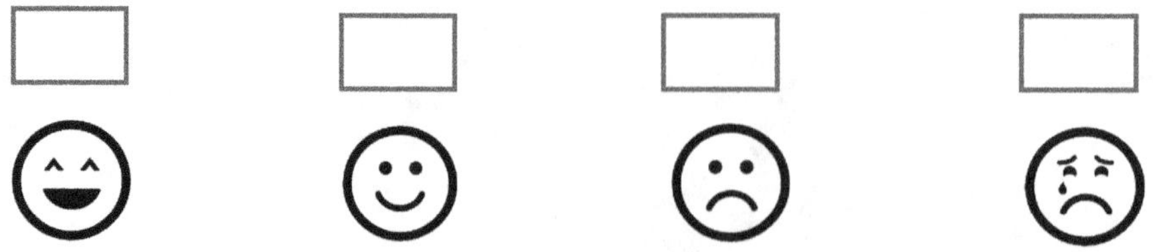

Grateful Thoughts

THIS WEEK I AM GRATEFUL FOR

I AM BLESSED TO HAVE THESE PEOPLE IN MY LIFE

5 REASONS TO BE THANKFUL

1.
2.
3.
4.
5.

NOTES:

Me Time

Write down the things that make you happy. Then, check the box every day that you spend time with that activity.

Activity	S	M	T	W	T	F	S
	☐	☐	☐	☐	☐	☐	☐
	☐	☐	☐	☐	☐	☐	☐
	☐	☐	☐	☐	☐	☐	☐
	☐	☐	☐	☐	☐	☐	☐
	☐	☐	☐	☐	☐	☐	☐
	☐	☐	☐	☐	☐	☐	☐
	☐	☐	☐	☐	☐	☐	☐
	☐	☐	☐	☐	☐	☐	☐

NOTES:

Self Care

DAILY **INSPIRATION**

WATER INTAKE:

FITNESS **GOALS**

One day at a time...

THANKFUL **FOR**

DAILY **MEALS**

BREAKFAST:

LUNCH:

DINNER:

SNACKS:

Personal Goals

MY SELF GOALS FOR THIS YEAR:

2 THINGS I CAN CHANGE TO MEET MY GOALS:

MY GREATEST OBSTACLE GOING FORWARD:

Good things take time

Mental Health Monitor

DAILY

_____
_____
_____
_____
_____
_____
_____
_____
_____
_____
_____
_____

WEEKLY

_____
_____
_____
_____
_____
_____
_____
_____
_____
_____
_____
_____

PERSONAL REFLECTIONS

Self Care Goals

TIME FRAME	MY GOALS	STEPS I'LL TAKE

be wild ~ be true ~ be happy

Self Care Techniques

MIND

_____
_____
_____
_____
_____
_____
_____
_____
_____
_____

BODY

_____
_____
_____
_____
_____
_____
_____
_____
_____
_____

PERSONAL REFLECTIONS

One Day at a Time

FEBRUARY

S	M	T	W	T	F	S
					1	2
3	4	5	6	7	8	9
10	11	12	13	14	15	16
17	18	19	20	21	22	23
24	25	26	27	28		

NOTES & REMINDERS

One Day at a Time

MONDAY'S **MOOD**

TUESDAY'S **MOOD**

WEDNESDAY'S **MOOD**

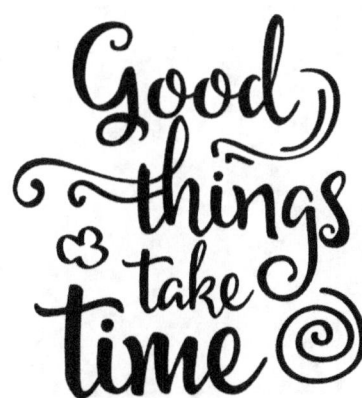

THURSDAY'S **MOOD**

One Day at a Time

FRIDAY'S MOOD

SATURDAY'S MOOD

SUNDAY'S MOOD

THOUGHTS & REFLECTIONS ABOUT THE PAST WEEK

Positive Thinking

SELF CARE TO DO LIST:

- [ ] _____
- [ ] _____
- [ ] _____
- [ ] _____
- [ ] _____
- [ ] _____
- [ ] _____
- [ ] _____
- [ ] _____
- [ ] _____
- [ ] _____
- [ ] _____
- [ ] _____
- [ ] _____
- [ ] _____

PHYSICAL NEEDS

EMOTIONAL NEEDS

HOW I FEEL TODAY

I WANT TO WORK ON...

Mood Meter

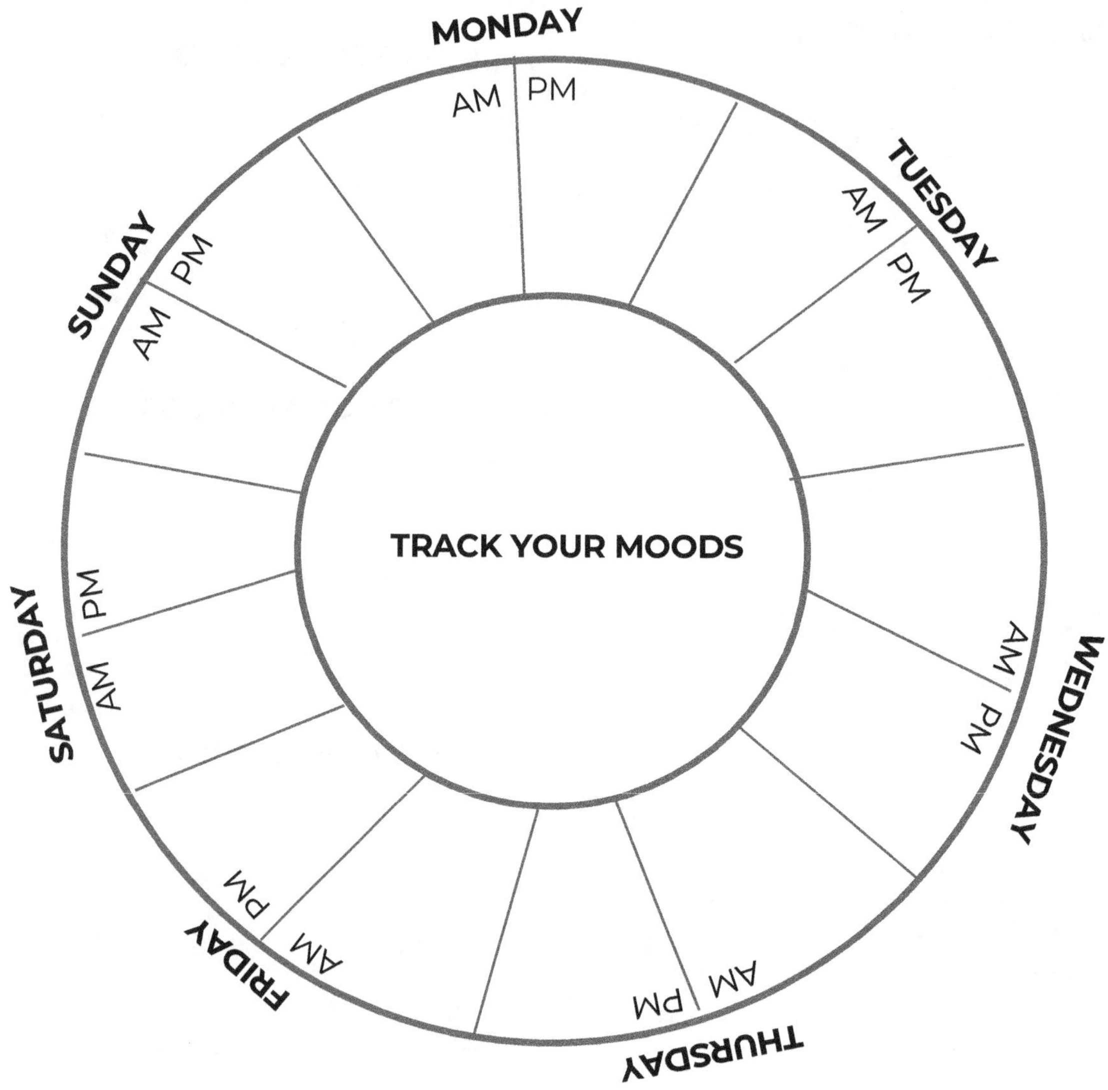
MONDAY
AM
PM
TUESDAY
AM
PM
WEDNESDAY
AM
PM
THURSDAY
AM
PM
FRIDAY
AM
PM
SATURDAY
AM
PM
SUNDAY
AM
PM
TRACK YOUR MOODS

COLOR SCALE

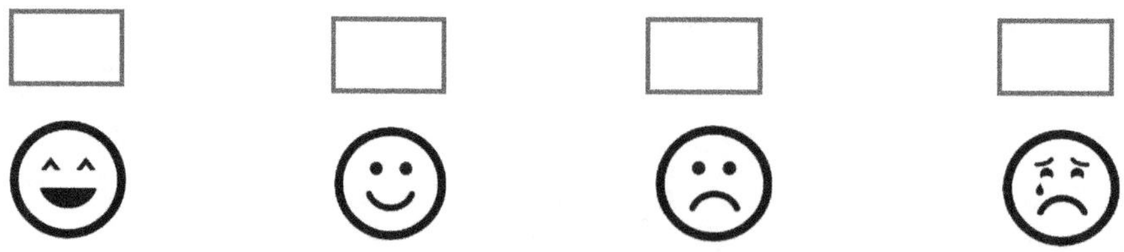

Self Care Log

HOW I CAN MINIMIZE THE NEGATIVITY IN MY LIFE

POSITIVE STEPS I CAN TAKE TO BE HAPPY

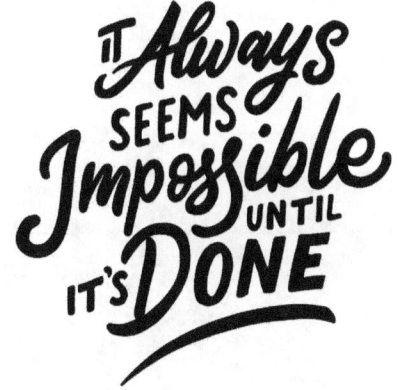

Grateful Thoughts

THIS WEEK I AM GRATEFUL FOR

I AM BLESSED TO HAVE THESE PEOPLE IN MY LIFE

5 REASONS TO BE THANKFUL

1.
2.
3.
4.
5.

NOTES:

Self Care

DAILY **INSPIRATION**

WATER INTAKE:

FITNESS **GOALS**

One day at a time...

THANKFUL **FOR**

DAILY **MEALS**

BREAKFAST:

LUNCH:

DINNER:

SNACKS:

Personal Goals

MY SELF GOALS FOR THIS YEAR:

2 THINGS I CAN CHANGE TO MEET MY GOALS:

MY GREATEST OBSTACLE GOING FORWARD:

Good things take time

Mental Health Monitor

DAILY

_____
_____
_____
_____
_____
_____
_____
_____
_____
_____
_____

WEEKLY

_____
_____
_____
_____
_____
_____
_____
_____
_____
_____
_____

PERSONAL REFLECTIONS

Self Care Goals

TIME FRAME	MY GOALS	STEPS I'LL TAKE

be wild ~ be true ~ be happy

One Day at a Time

MARCH

S	M	T	W	T	F	S
					1	2
3	4	5	6	7	8	9
10	11	12	13	14	15	16
17	18	19	20	21	22	23
24	25	26	27	28	29	30
31						

NOTES & REMINDERS

One Day at a Time

MONDAY'S MOOD

TUESDAY'S MOOD

WEDNESDAY'S MOOD

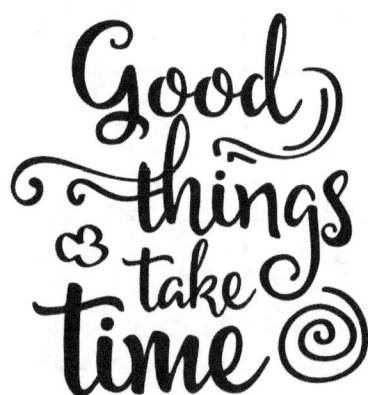

THURSDAY'S MOOD

One Day at a Time

FRIDAY'S MOOD

SATURDAY'S MOOD

SUNDAY'S MOOD

THOUGHTS & REFLECTIONS ABOUT THE PAST WEEK

Positive Thinking

SELF CARE TO DO LIST:

- [ ] _____
- [ ] _____
- [ ] _____
- [ ] _____
- [ ] _____
- [ ] _____
- [ ] _____
- [ ] _____
- [ ] _____
- [ ] _____
- [ ] _____
- [ ] _____
- [ ] _____
- [ ] _____

PHYSICAL NEEDS

EMOTIONAL NEEDS

HOW I FEEL TODAY

I WANT TO WORK ON...

Mood Meter

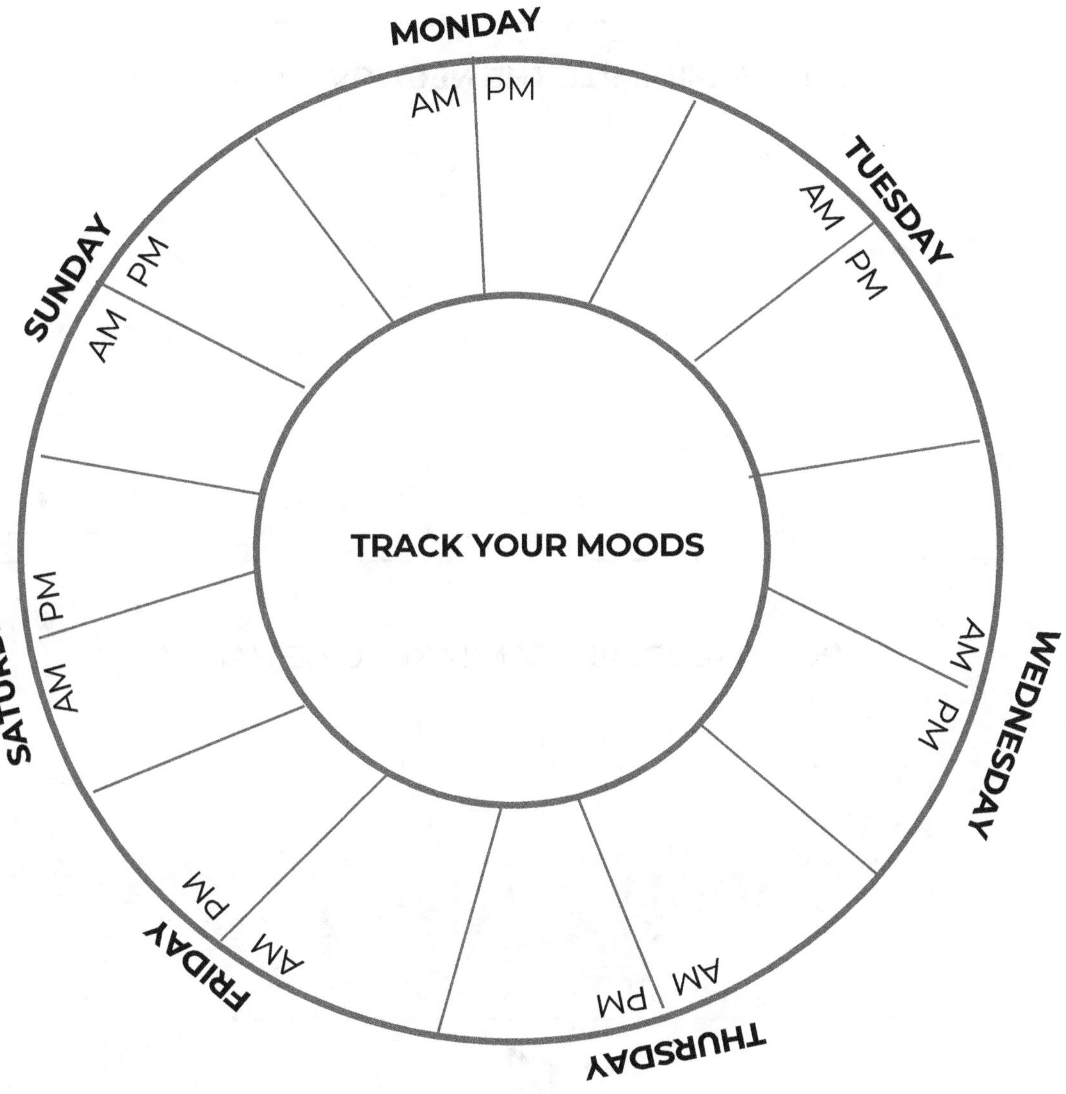

MONDAY
AM | PM

TUESDAY
AM | PM

WEDNESDAY
AM | PM

THURSDAY
AM | PM

FRIDAY
AM | PM

SATURDAY
AM | PM

SUNDAY
AM | PM

TRACK YOUR MOODS

COLOR SCALE

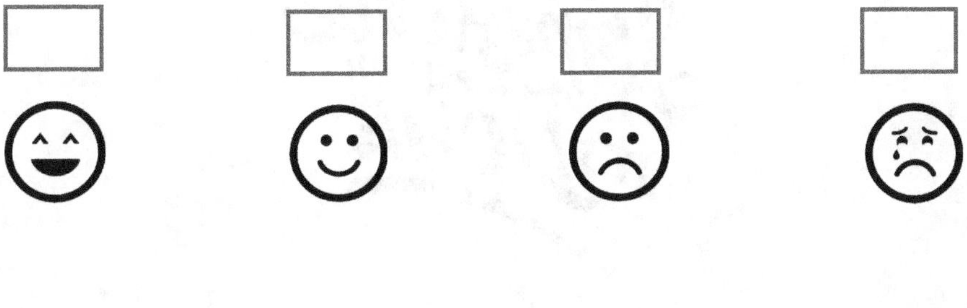

Self Care Log

HOW I CAN MINIMIZE THE NEGATIVITY IN MY LIFE

POSITIVE STEPS I CAN TAKE TO BE HAPPY

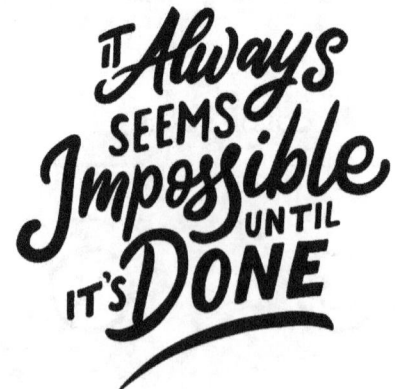

Grateful Thoughts

THIS WEEK I AM GRATEFUL FOR

I AM BLESSED TO HAVE THESE PEOPLE IN MY LIFE

5 REASONS TO BE THANKFUL

1
2
3
4
5

NOTES:

Me Time

Write down the things that make you happy. Then, check the box every day that you spend time with that activity.

NOTES:

Self Care

DAILY **INSPIRATION**

WATER INTAKE:

FITNESS **GOALS**

One day at a time...

THANKFUL **FOR**

DAILY **MEALS**

BREAKFAST:

LUNCH:

DINNER:

SNACKS:

Personal Goals

MY SELF GOALS FOR THIS YEAR:

2 THINGS I CAN CHANGE TO MEET MY GOALS:

MY GREATEST OBSTACLE GOING FORWARD:

Good things take time

Mental Health Monitor

DAILY

WEEKLY

PERSONAL REFLECTIONS

Self Care Goals

TIME FRAME	MY GOALS	STEPS I'LL TAKE

be wild ~ be true ~ be happy

Self Care Techniques

MIND

_____
_____
_____
_____
_____
_____
_____
_____
_____
_____
_____
_____

BODY

_____
_____
_____
_____
_____
_____
_____
_____
_____
_____
_____
_____

PERSONAL REFLECTIONS

One Day at a Time

APRIL

S	M	T	W	T	F	S
	1	2	3	4	5	6
7	8	9	10	11	12	13
14	15	16	17	18	19	20
21	22	23	24	25	26	27
28	29	30				

NOTES & REMINDERS

One Day at a Time

MONDAY'S **MOOD**

TUESDAY'S **MOOD**

WEDNESDAY'S **MOOD**

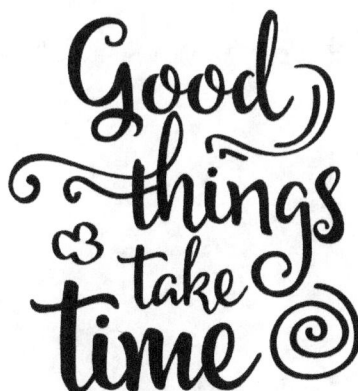

THURSDAY'S **MOOD**

One Day at a Time

FRIDAY'S MOOD

SATURDAY'S MOOD

SUNDAY'S MOOD

THOUGHTS & REFLECTIONS ABOUT THE PAST WEEK

Mood Meter

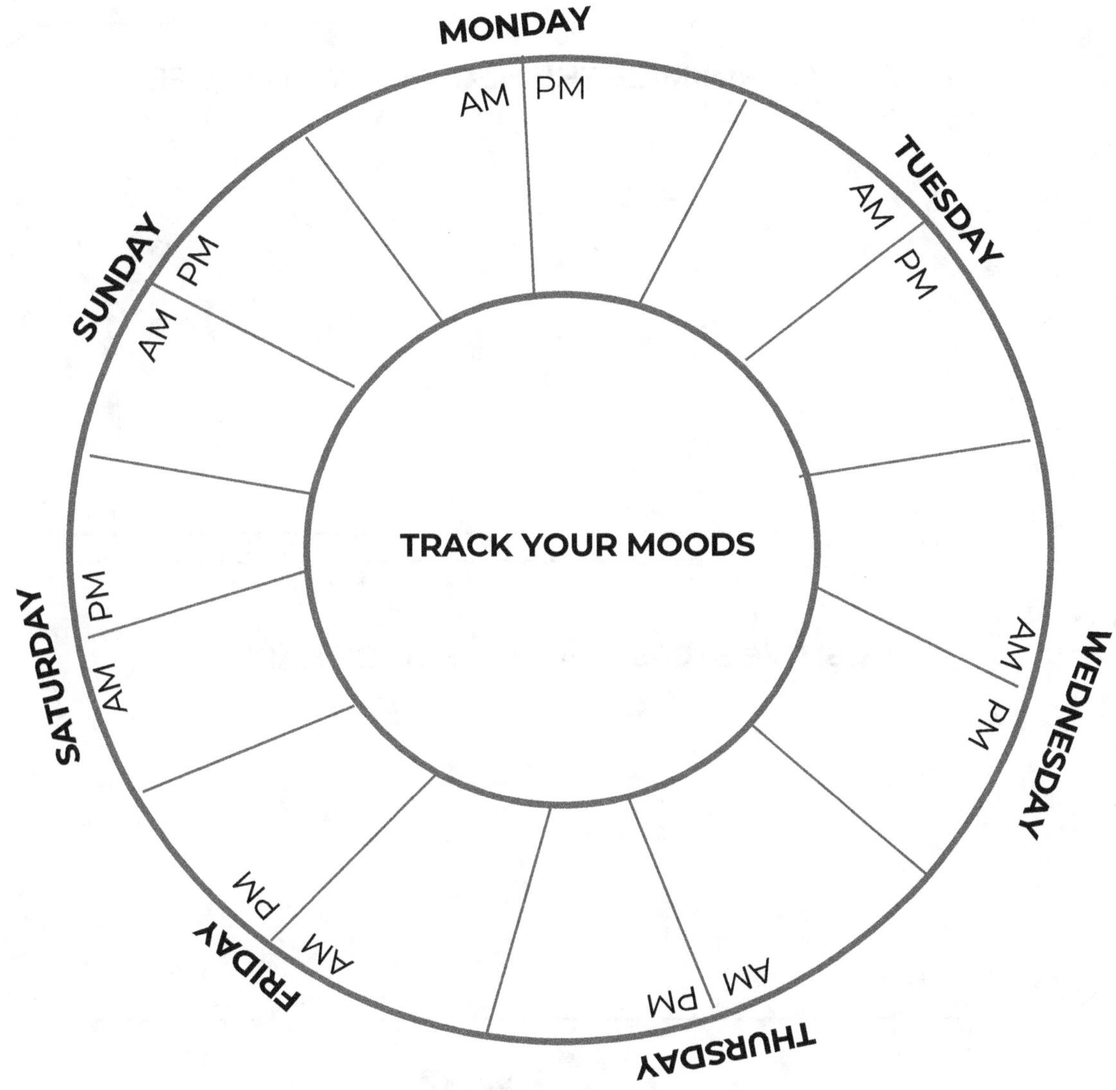

MONDAY — AM | PM
TUESDAY — AM | PM
WEDNESDAY — AM | PM
THURSDAY — AM | PM
FRIDAY — AM | PM
SATURDAY — AM | PM
SUNDAY — AM | PM

TRACK YOUR MOODS

COLOR SCALE

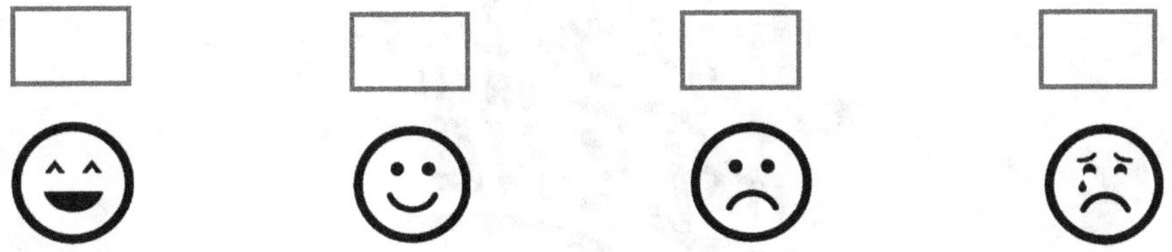

Self Care Log

HOW I CAN MINIMIZE THE NEGATIVITY IN MY LIFE

POSITIVE STEPS I CAN TAKE TO BE HAPPY

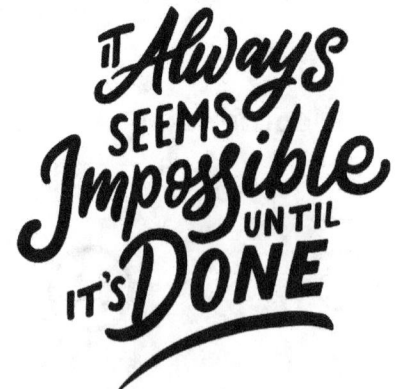

Grateful Thoughts

THIS WEEK I AM GRATEFUL FOR

I AM BLESSED TO HAVE THESE PEOPLE IN MY LIFE

5 REASONS TO BE THANKFUL

1.
2.
3.
4.
5.

NOTES:

Self Care

DAILY **INSPIRATION**

WATER INTAKE:

FITNESS **GOALS**

One day at a time...

THANKFUL **FOR**

DAILY **MEALS**

BREAKFAST:

LUNCH:

DINNER:

SNACKS:

Personal Goals

MY SELF GOALS FOR THIS YEAR:

2 THINGS I CAN CHANGE TO MEET MY GOALS:

MY GREATEST OBSTACLE GOING FORWARD:

Good things take time

Mental Health Monitor

DAILY

_____
_____
_____
_____
_____
_____
_____
_____
_____
_____
_____
_____

WEEKLY

_____
_____
_____
_____
_____
_____
_____
_____
_____
_____
_____
_____

PERSONAL REFLECTIONS

Self Care Goals

TIME FRAME	MY GOALS	STEPS I'LL TAKE

be wild ~ be true ~ be happy

Self Care Techniques

MIND   **BODY**

PERSONAL REFLECTIONS

One Day at a Time

MAY

S	M	T	W	T	F	S
			1	2	3	4
5	6	7	8	9	10	11
12	13	14	15	16	17	18
19	20	21	22	23	24	25
26	27	28	29	30	31	

NOTES & REMINDERS

One Day at a Time

MONDAY'S MOOD

TUESDAY'S MOOD

WEDNESDAY'S MOOD

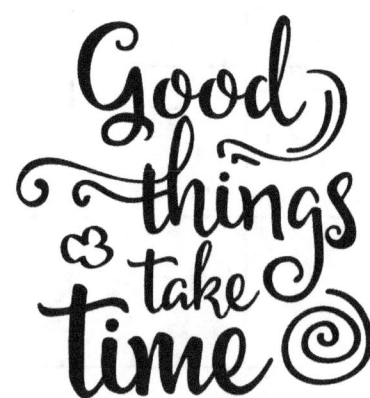

THURSDAY'S MOOD

One Day at a Time

FRIDAY'S **MOOD**

SATURDAY'S **MOOD**

SUNDAY'S **MOOD**

THOUGHTS & REFLECTIONS ABOUT THE PAST WEEK

My Mood Today

DRAWING THAT DESCRIBES YOUR **FEELINGS**

It's just a bad day, Not a bad life

Positive Thinking

SELF CARE TO DO LIST:

- [ ] _____
- [ ] _____
- [ ] _____
- [ ] _____
- [ ] _____
- [ ] _____
- [ ] _____
- [ ] _____
- [ ] _____
- [ ] _____
- [ ] _____
- [ ] _____
- [ ] _____
- [ ] _____

PHYSICAL NEEDS

EMOTIONAL NEEDS

HOW I FEEL TODAY

I WANT TO WORK ON...

Mood Meter

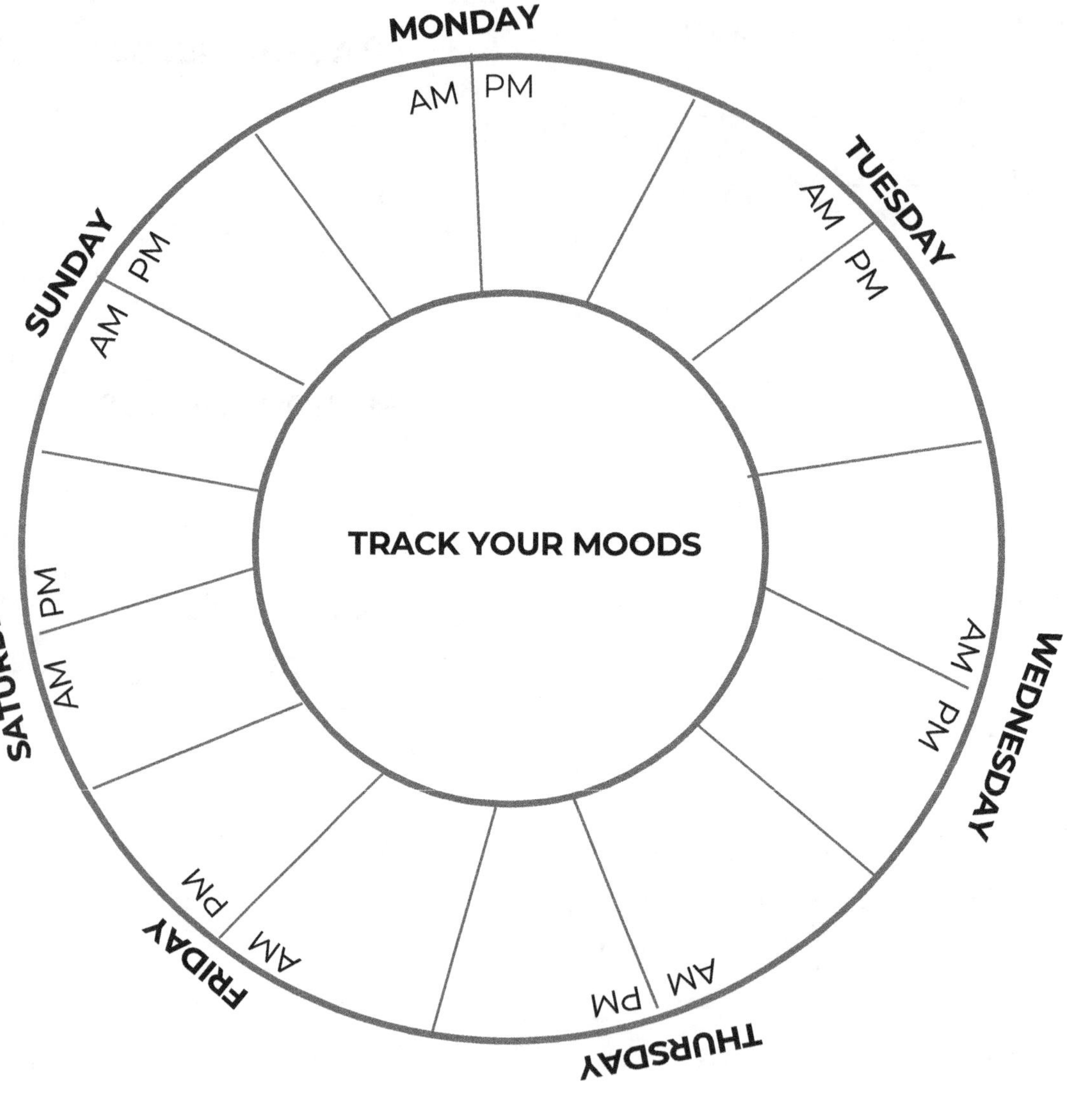
MONDAY
AM
PM
TUESDAY
AM
PM
WEDNESDAY
AM
PM
THURSDAY
AM
PM
FRIDAY
AM
PM
SATURDAY
AM
PM
SUNDAY
AM
PM
TRACK YOUR MOODS

COLOR SCALE

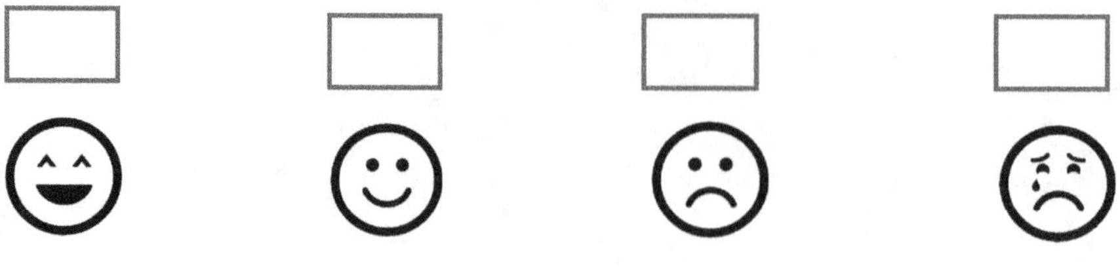

Self Care Log

HOW I CAN **MINIMIZE THE NEGATIVITY** IN MY LIFE

POSITIVE STEPS I CAN TAKE TO BE HAPPY

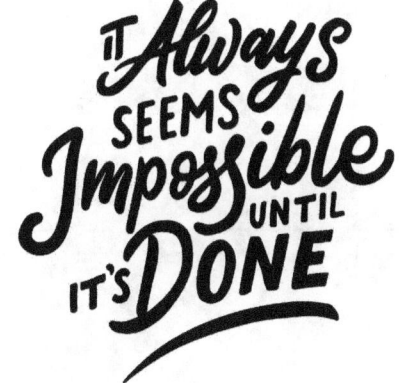

Grateful Thoughts

THIS WEEK I AM GRATEFUL FOR

I AM BLESSED TO HAVE THESE PEOPLE IN MY LIFE

5 REASONS TO BE THANKFUL

1
2
3
4
5

NOTES:

Me Time

Write down the things that make you happy. Then, check the box every day that you spend time with that activity.

NOTES:

Self Care

DAILY INSPIRATION

WATER INTAKE:

FITNESS GOALS

One day at a time...

THANKFUL FOR

DAILY MEALS

BREAKFAST:

LUNCH:

DINNER:

SNACKS:

Personal Goals

MY SELF GOALS FOR THIS YEAR:

2 THINGS I CAN CHANGE TO MEET MY GOALS:

MY GREATEST OBSTACLE GOING FORWARD:

Good things take time

Mental Health Monitor

DAILY

_____
_____
_____
_____
_____
_____
_____
_____
_____
_____

WEEKLY

_____
_____
_____
_____
_____
_____
_____
_____
_____
_____

PERSONAL REFLECTIONS

Self Care Goals

TIME FRAME	MY GOALS	STEPS I'LL TAKE

be wild ~ be true ~ be happy

Self Care Techniques

MIND

BODY

PERSONAL REFLECTIONS

One Day at a Time

JUNE

S	M	T	W	T	F	S
						1
2	3	4	5	6	7	8
9	10	11	12	13	14	15
16	17	18	19	20	21	22
23	24	25	26	27	28	29
30						

NOTES & REMINDERS

One Day at a Time

MONDAY'S MOOD

TUESDAY'S MOOD

WEDNESDAY'S MOOD

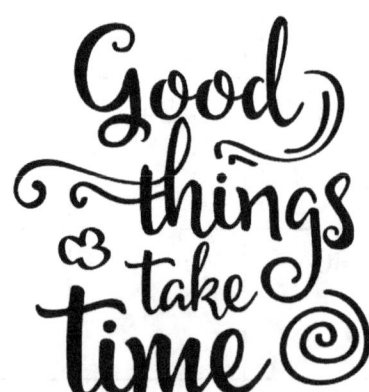

THURSDAY'S MOOD

One Day at a Time

FRIDAY'S MOOD

SATURDAY'S MOOD

SUNDAY'S MOOD

THOUGHTS & REFLECTIONS ABOUT THE PAST WEEK

Positive Thinking

SELF CARE TO DO LIST:

- [ ] _____
- [ ] _____
- [ ] _____
- [ ] _____
- [ ] _____
- [ ] _____
- [ ] _____
- [ ] _____
- [ ] _____
- [ ] _____
- [ ] _____
- [ ] _____
- [ ] _____
- [ ] _____

PHYSICAL NEEDS

EMOTIONAL NEEDS

HOW I FEEL TODAY

I WANT TO WORK ON...

Mood Meter

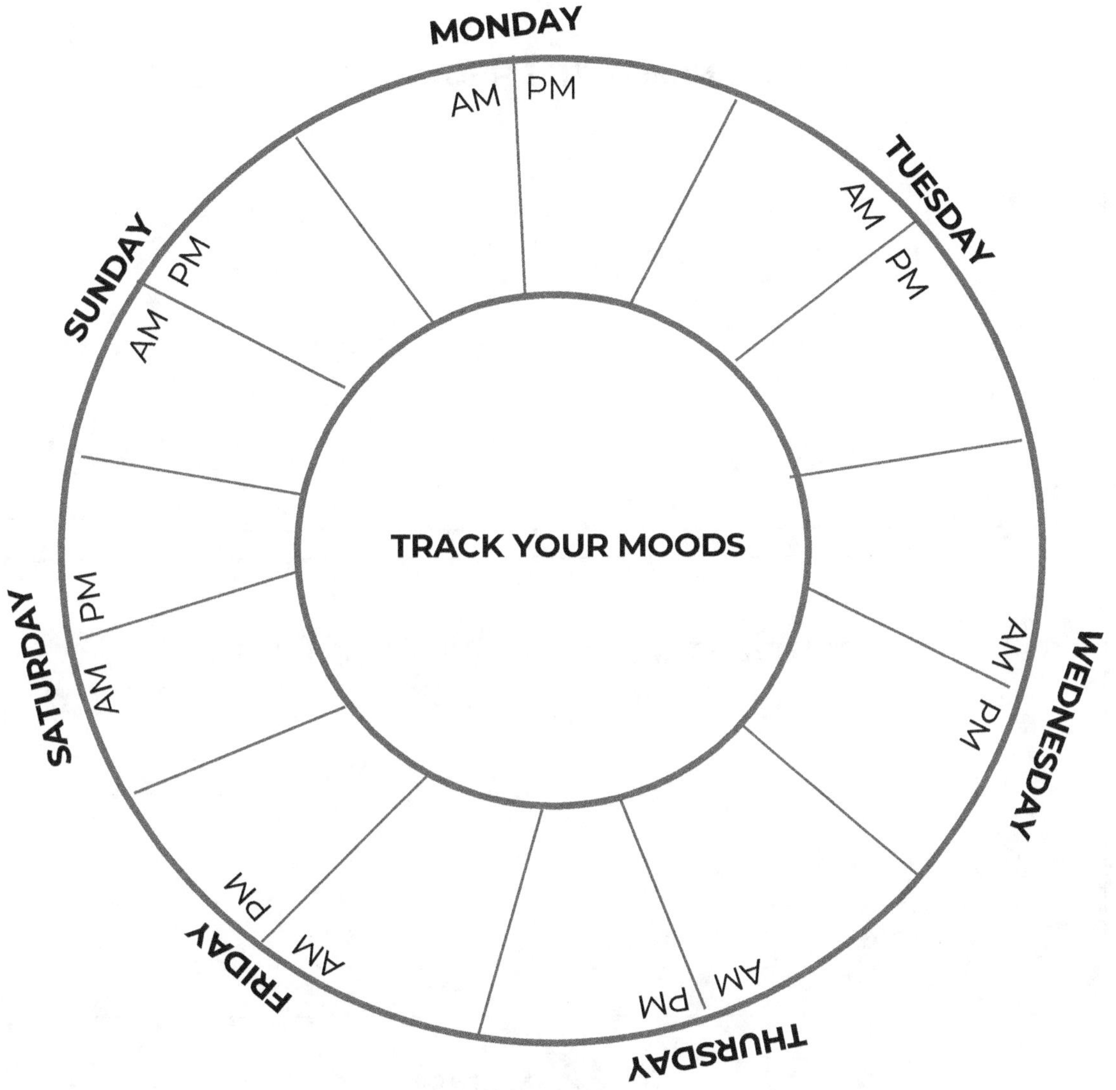
MONDAY
AM
PM
TUESDAY
AM
PM
WEDNESDAY
AM
PM
THURSDAY
AM
PM
FRIDAY
AM
PM
SATURDAY
AM
PM
SUNDAY
AM
PM
TRACK YOUR MOODS

COLOR SCALE

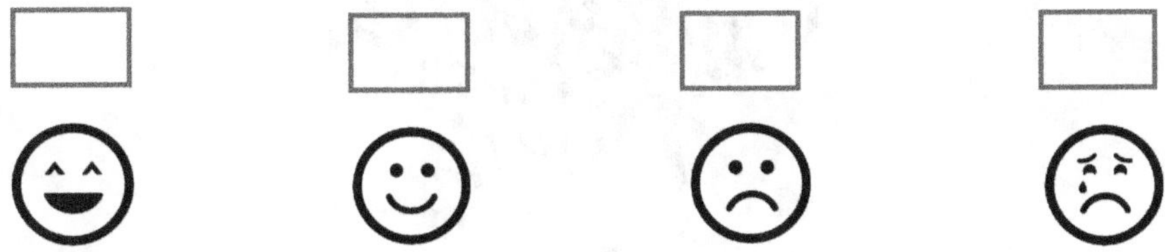

Self Care Log

HOW I CAN MINIMIZE THE NEGATIVITY IN MY LIFE

POSITIVE STEPS I CAN TAKE TO BE HAPPY

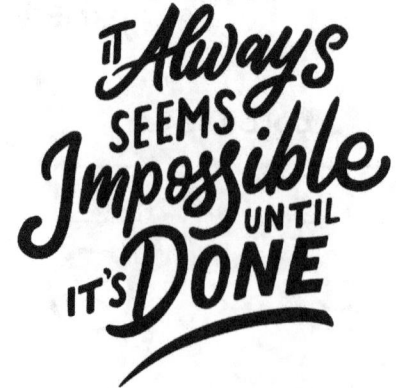

Grateful Thoughts

THIS WEEK I AM GRATEFUL FOR

I AM BLESSED TO HAVE THESE PEOPLE IN MY LIFE

5 REASONS TO BE THANKFUL

1.
2.
3.
4.
5.

NOTES:

Me Time

Write down the things that make you happy. Then, check the box every day that you spend time with that activity.

NOTES:

Self Care

DAILY **INSPIRATION**

WATER INTAKE:

FITNESS **GOALS**

One day at a time...

THANKFUL **FOR**

DAILY **MEALS**

BREAKFAST:

LUNCH:

DINNER:

SNACKS:

Personal Goals

MY SELF GOALS FOR THIS YEAR:

2 THINGS I CAN CHANGE TO MEET MY GOALS:

MY GREATEST OBSTACLE GOING FORWARD:

Good things take time

Mental Health Monitor

DAILY

_____
_____
_____
_____
_____
_____
_____
_____
_____
_____
_____
_____

WEEKLY

_____
_____
_____
_____
_____
_____
_____
_____
_____
_____
_____
_____

PERSONAL REFLECTIONS

Self Care Goals

TIME FRAME	MY GOALS	STEPS I'LL TAKE

be wild ~ be true ~ be happy

Self Care Techniques

MIND

_____
_____
_____
_____
_____
_____
_____
_____
_____
_____
_____

BODY

_____
_____
_____
_____
_____
_____
_____
_____
_____
_____
_____

PERSONAL REFLECTIONS

One Day at a Time

JULY

S	M	T	W	T	F	S
	1	2	3	4	5	6
7	8	9	10	11	12	13
14	15	16	17	18	19	20
21	22	23	24	25	26	27
28	29	30	31			

NOTES & REMINDERS

One Day at a Time

MONDAY'S MOOD

TUESDAY'S MOOD

WEDNESDAY'S MOOD

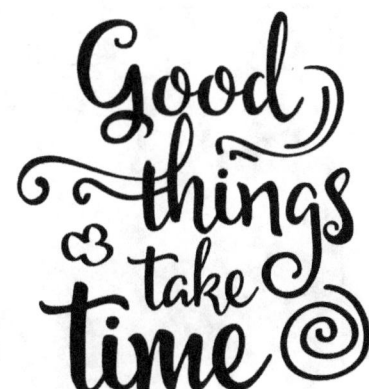

THURSDAY'S MOOD

One Day at a Time

FRIDAY'S MOOD

SATURDAY'S MOOD

SUNDAY'S MOOD

THOUGHTS & REFLECTIONS ABOUT THE PAST WEEK

Positive Thinking

SELF CARE TO DO LIST:

- [ ] _____
- [ ] _____
- [ ] _____
- [ ] _____
- [ ] _____
- [ ] _____
- [ ] _____
- [ ] _____
- [ ] _____
- [ ] _____
- [ ] _____
- [ ] _____
- [ ] _____
- [ ] _____

PHYSICAL NEEDS

EMOTIONAL NEEDS

HOW I FEEL TODAY

I WANT TO WORK ON...

Mood Meter

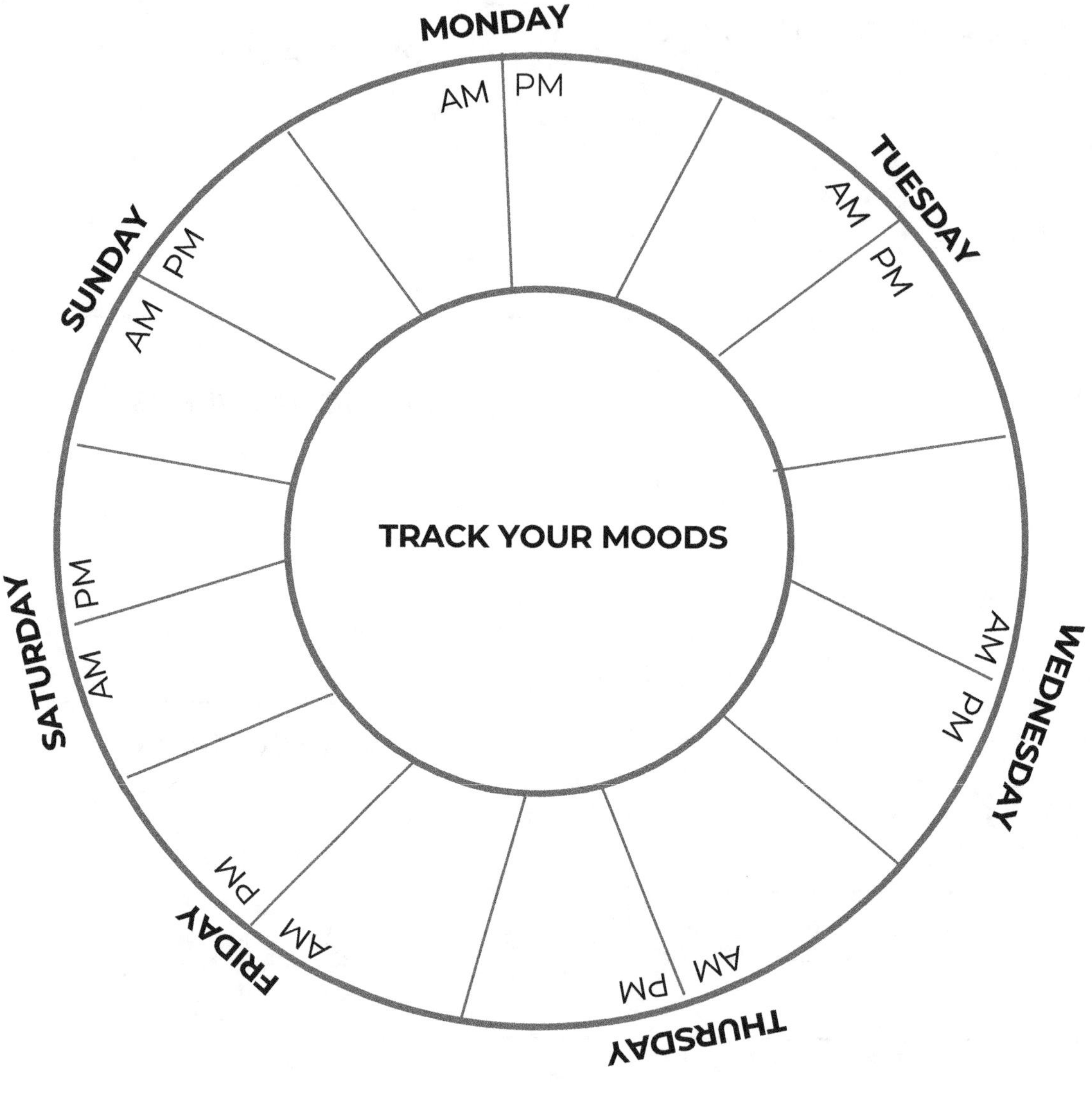

MONDAY
AM
PM
TUESDAY
AM
PM
WEDNESDAY
AM
PM
THURSDAY
AM
PM
FRIDAY
AM
PM
SATURDAY
AM
PM
SUNDAY
AM
PM
TRACK YOUR MOODS

COLOR SCALE

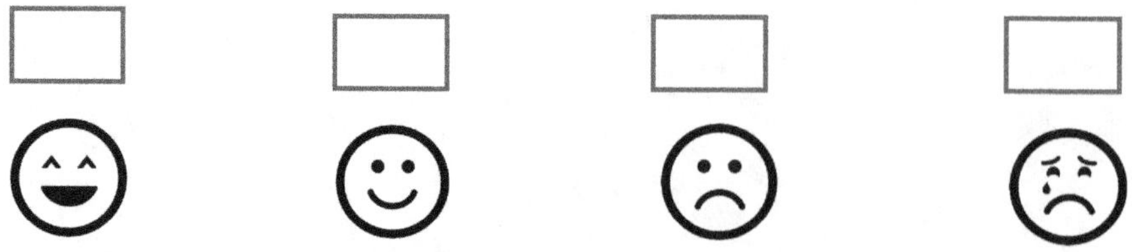

Self Care Log

HOW I CAN **MINIMIZE THE NEGATIVITY** IN MY LIFE

POSITIVE STEPS I CAN TAKE TO BE HAPPY

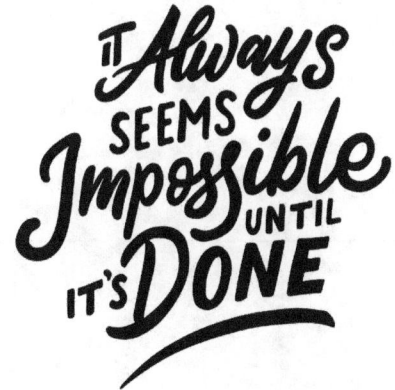

Grateful Thoughts

THIS WEEK I AM GRATEFUL FOR

I AM BLESSED TO HAVE THESE PEOPLE IN MY LIFE

5 REASONS TO BE THANKFUL

1.
2.
3.
4.
5.

NOTES:

Me Time

Write down the things that make you happy. Then, check the box every day that you spend time with that activity.

NOTES:

Self Care

DAILY **INSIGHT**

DAILY **MEALS**

BREAKFAST:

_____
_____
_____

WATER INTAKE:

▯ ▯ ▯ ▯ ▯ ▯ ▯ ▯

LUNCH:

_____
_____
_____

FITNESS **GOALS**

_____
_____
_____

DINNER:

_____
_____
_____

One day at a time...

SNACKS:

THANKFUL **FOR**

_____
_____
_____
_____
_____

Personal Goals

MY SELF GOALS FOR THIS YEAR:

2 THINGS I CAN CHANGE TO MEET MY GOALS:

MY GREATEST OBSTACLE GOING FORWARD:

Good things take time

Mental Health Monitor

DAILY

_____
_____
_____
_____
_____
_____
_____
_____
_____
_____
_____
_____

WEEKLY

_____
_____
_____
_____
_____
_____
_____
_____
_____
_____
_____
_____

PERSONAL REFLECTIONS

Self Care Goals

TIME FRAME	MY GOALS	STEPS I'LL TAKE

be wild ~ be true ~ be happy

Self Care Techniques

MIND

BODY

PERSONAL REFLECTIONS

One Day at a Time

AUGUST

S	M	T	W	T	F	S
				1	2	3
4	5	6	7	8	9	10
11	12	13	14	15	16	17
18	19	20	21	22	23	24
25	26	27	28	29	30	31

NOTES & REMINDERS

One Day at a Time

MONDAY'S MOOD

TUESDAY'S MOOD

WEDNESDAY'S MOOD

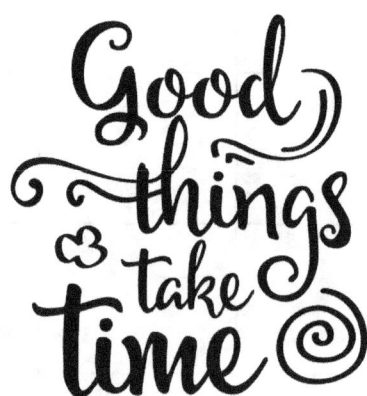

THURSDAY'S MOOD

One Day at a Time

FRIDAY'S MOOD

SATURDAY'S MOOD

SUNDAY'S MOOD

THOUGHTS & REFLECTIONS ABOUT THE PAST WEEK

Positive Thinking

SELF CARE TO DO LIST:

- [ ] _____
- [ ] _____
- [ ] _____
- [ ] _____
- [ ] _____
- [ ] _____
- [ ] _____
- [ ] _____
- [ ] _____
- [ ] _____
- [ ] _____
- [ ] _____
- [ ] _____
- [ ] _____

PHYSICAL NEEDS

EMOTIONAL NEEDS

HOW I FEEL TODAY

I WANT TO WORK ON...

Mood Meter

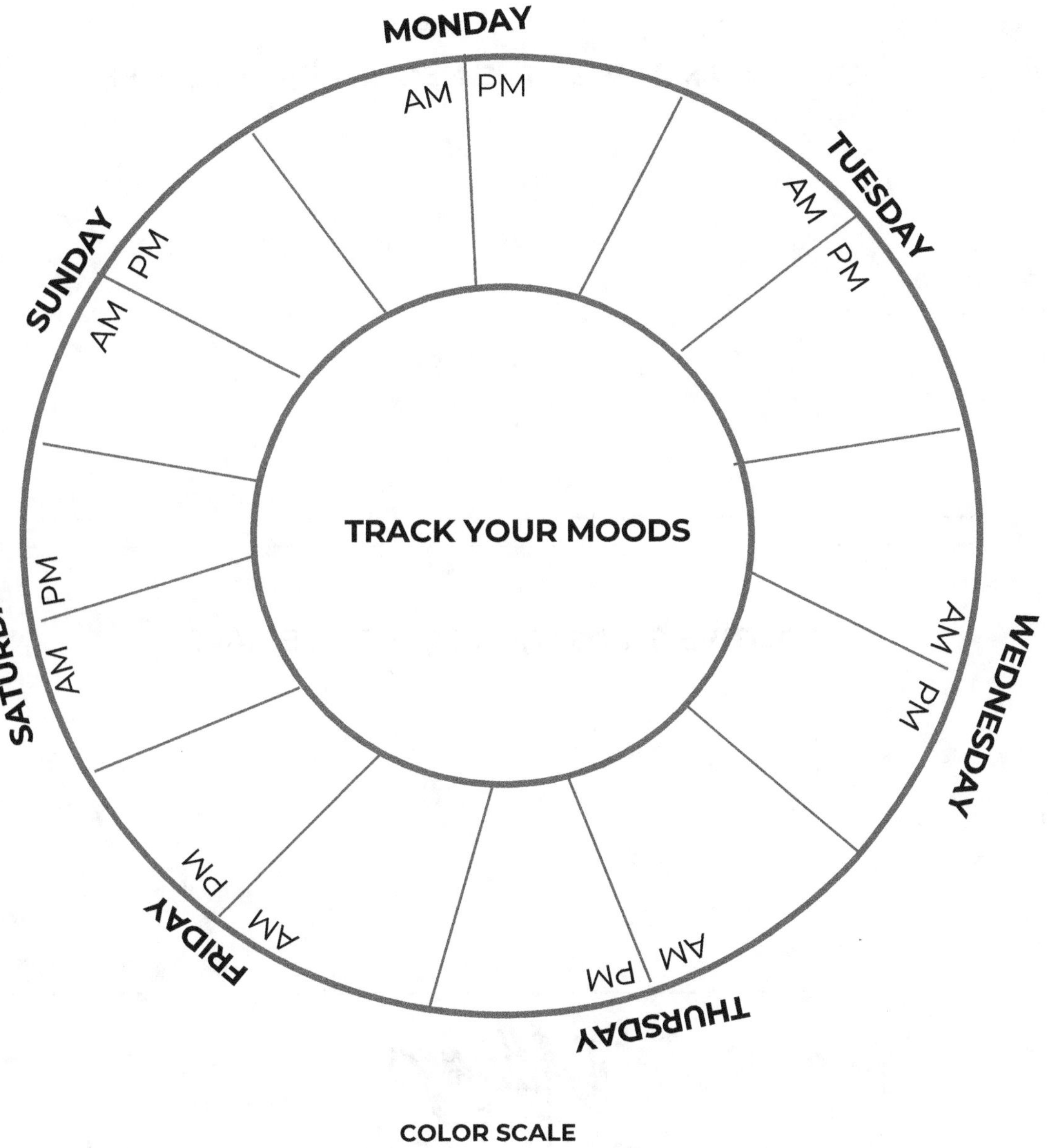

MONDAY
AM | PM

TUESDAY
AM | PM

WEDNESDAY
AM | PM

THURSDAY
AM | PM

FRIDAY
AM | PM

SATURDAY
AM | PM

SUNDAY
AM | PM

TRACK YOUR MOODS

COLOR SCALE

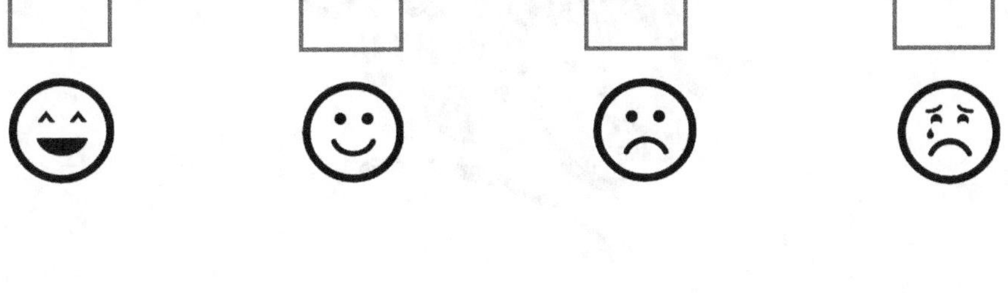

Self Care Log

HOW I CAN **MINIMIZE THE NEGATIVITY** IN MY LIFE

POSITIVE STEPS I CAN TAKE TO BE HAPPY

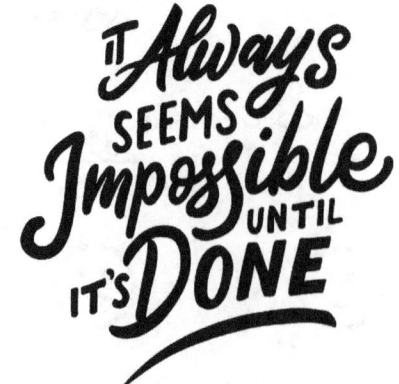

Grateful Thoughts

THIS WEEK I AM GRATEFUL FOR

I AM BLESSED TO HAVE THESE PEOPLE IN MY LIFE

5 REASONS TO BE THANKFUL

1
2
3
4
5

NOTES:

Me Time

Write down the things that make you happy. Then, check the box every day that you spend time with that activity.

NOTES:

Self Care

DAILY **INSPIRATION**

WATER INTAKE:

FITNESS **GOALS**

One day at a time...

THANKFUL **FOR**

DAILY **MEALS**

BREAKFAST:

LUNCH:

DINNER:

SNACKS:

Personal Goals

MY SELF GOALS FOR THIS YEAR:

2 THINGS I CAN CHANGE TO MEET MY GOALS:

MY GREATEST OBSTACLE GOING FORWARD:

Good things take time

Mental Health Monitor

DAILY

_____
_____
_____
_____
_____
_____
_____
_____
_____
_____
_____
_____

WEEKLY

_____
_____
_____
_____
_____
_____
_____
_____
_____
_____
_____
_____

PERSONAL REFLECTIONS

Self Care Goals

TIME FRAME	MY GOALS	STEPS I'LL TAKE

be wild ~ be true ~ be happy

Self Care Techniques

MIND

_____
_____
_____
_____
_____
_____
_____
_____
_____
_____

BODY

_____
_____
_____
_____
_____
_____
_____
_____
_____
_____

PERSONAL REFLECTIONS

One Day at a Time

SEPTEMBER

S	M	T	W	T	F	S
1	2	3	4	5	6	7
8	9	10	11	12	13	14
15	16	17	18	19	20	21
22	23	24	25	26	27	28
29	30					

NOTES & REMINDERS

One Day at a Time

MONDAY'S **MOOD**

TUESDAY'S **MOOD**

WEDNESDAY'S **MOOD**

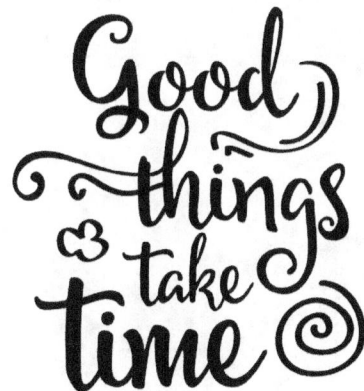

THURSDAY'S **MOOD**

One Day at a Time

FRIDAY'S MOOD

SATURDAY'S MOOD

SUNDAY'S MOOD

THOUGHTS & REFLECTIONS ABOUT THE PAST WEEK

Positive Thinking

SELF CARE TO DO LIST:

- [ ] _____
- [ ] _____
- [ ] _____
- [ ] _____
- [ ] _____
- [ ] _____
- [ ] _____
- [ ] _____
- [ ] _____
- [ ] _____
- [ ] _____
- [ ] _____
- [ ] _____
- [ ] _____

PHYSICAL NEEDS

EMOTIONAL NEEDS

HOW I FEEL TODAY

I WANT TO WORK ON...

Mood Meter

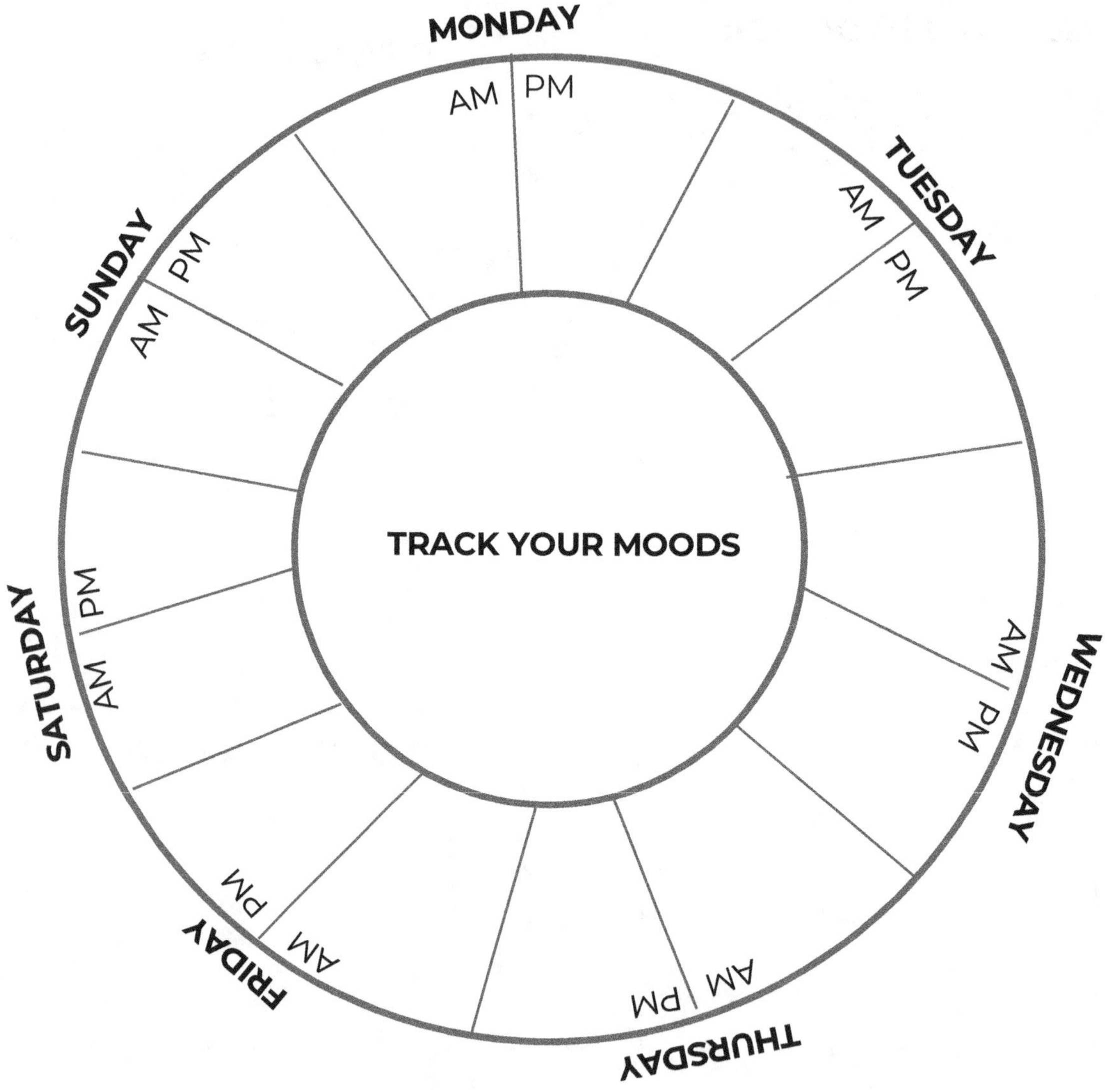

MONDAY

AM | PM

TUESDAY

AM | PM

WEDNESDAY

AM | PM

THURSDAY

AM | PM

FRIDAY

AM | PM

SATURDAY

AM | PM

SUNDAY

AM | PM

TRACK YOUR MOODS

COLOR SCALE

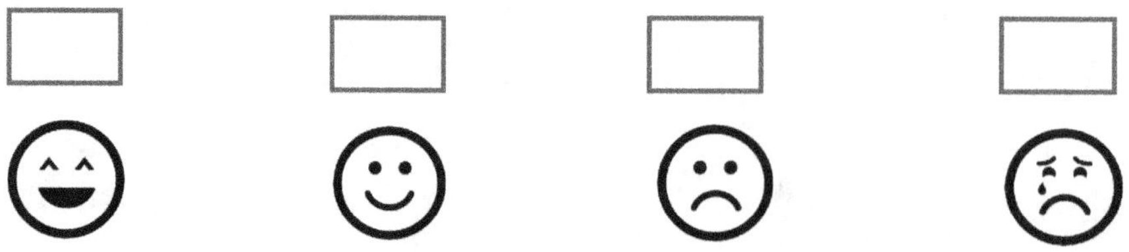

Self Care Log

HOW I CAN MINIMIZE THE NEGATIVITY IN MY LIFE

POSITIVE STEPS I CAN TAKE TO BE HAPPY

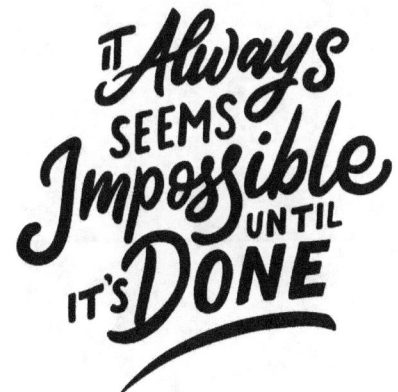

Grateful Thoughts

THIS WEEK I AM GRATEFUL FOR

I AM BLESSED TO HAVE THESE PEOPLE IN MY LIFE

5 REASONS TO BE THANKFUL

1
2
3
4
5

NOTES:

Me Time

Write down the things that make you happy. Then, check the box every day that you spend time with that activity.

NOTES:

Self Care

DAILY INSPIRATION

WATER INTAKE:

FITNESS GOALS

One day at a time...

THANKFUL FOR

DAILY MEALS

BREAKFAST:

LUNCH:

DINNER:

SNACKS:

Personal Goals

MY SELF GOALS FOR THIS YEAR:

2 THINGS I CAN CHANGE TO MEET MY GOALS:

MY GREATEST OBSTACLE GOING FORWARD:

Good things take time

Mental Health Monitor

DAILY

_____
_____
_____
_____
_____
_____
_____
_____
_____
_____

WEEKLY

_____
_____
_____
_____
_____
_____
_____
_____
_____
_____

PERSONAL REFLECTIONS

Self Care Goals

TIME FRAME	MY GOALS	STEPS I'LL TAKE

be wild — be true — be happy

Self Care Techniques

MIND

_____
_____
_____
_____
_____
_____
_____
_____
_____
_____
_____
_____

BODY

_____
_____
_____
_____
_____
_____
_____
_____
_____
_____
_____
_____

PERSONAL REFLECTIONS

One Day at a Time

OCTOBER

S	M	T	W	T	F	S
		1	2	3	4	5
6	7	8	9	10	11	12
13	14	15	16	17	18	19
20	21	22	23	24	25	26
27	28	29	30	31		

NOTES & REMINDERS

One Day at a Time

MONDAY'S MOOD

TUESDAY'S MOOD

WEDNESDAY'S MOOD

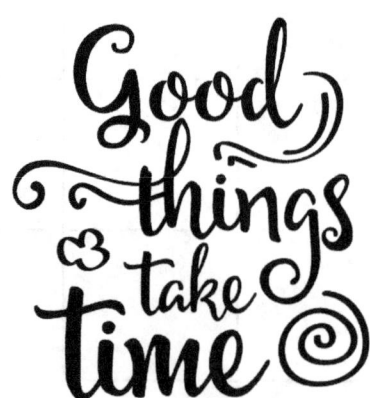

THURSDAY'S MOOD

One Day at a Time

FRIDAY'S **MOOD**

SATURDAY'S **MOOD**

SUNDAY'S **MOOD**

THOUGHTS & REFLECTIONS ABOUT THE PAST WEEK

Positive Thinking

SELF CARE TO DO LIST:

- [ ] _____
- [ ] _____
- [ ] _____
- [ ] _____
- [ ] _____
- [ ] _____
- [ ] _____
- [ ] _____
- [ ] _____
- [ ] _____
- [ ] _____
- [ ] _____
- [ ] _____
- [ ] _____

PHYSICAL NEEDS

EMOTIONAL NEEDS

HOW I FEEL TODAY

I WANT TO WORK ON...

Mood Meter

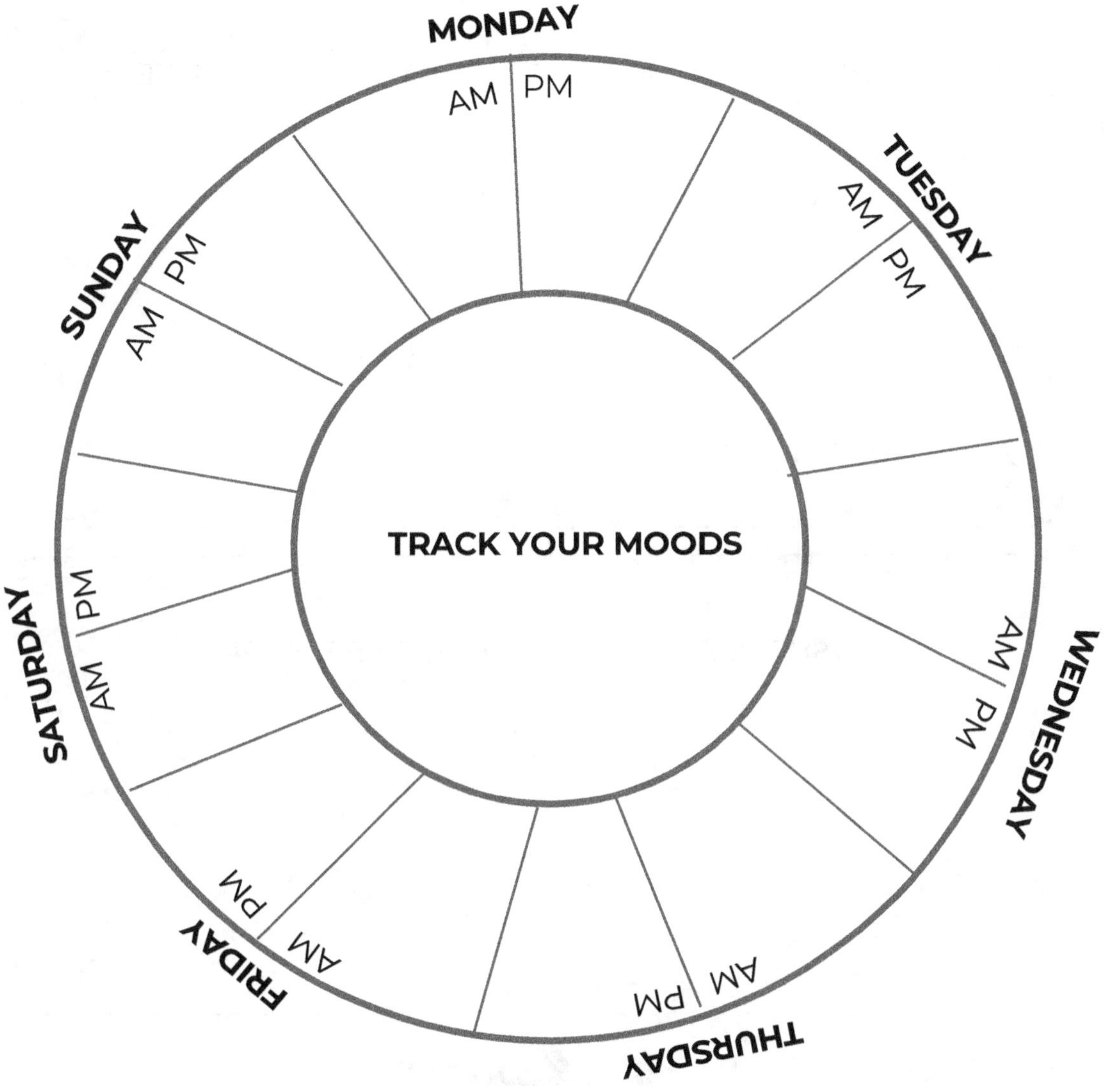

MONDAY — AM | PM
TUESDAY — AM | PM
WEDNESDAY — AM | PM
THURSDAY — AM | PM
FRIDAY — AM | PM
SATURDAY — AM | PM
SUNDAY — AM | PM

TRACK YOUR MOODS

COLOR SCALE

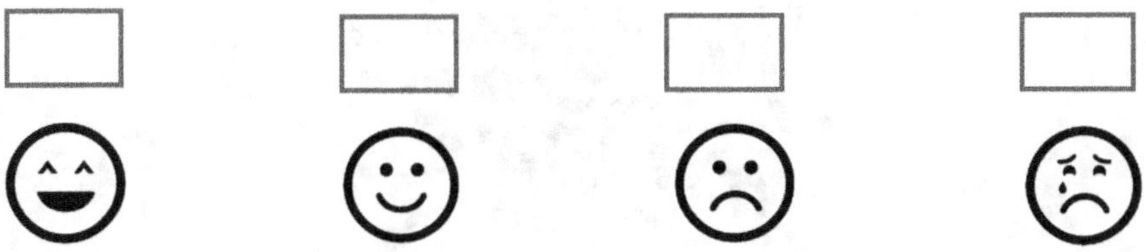

Self Care Log

HOW I CAN MINIMIZE THE NEGATIVITY IN MY LIFE

POSITIVE STEPS I CAN TAKE TO BE HAPPY

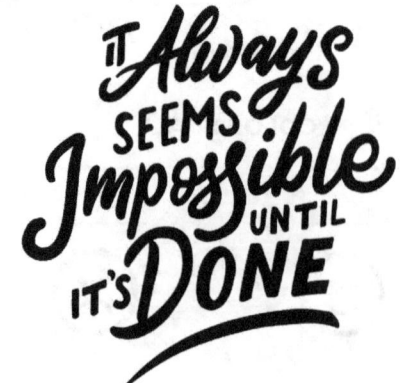

Grateful Thoughts

THIS WEEK I AM GRATEFUL FOR

I AM BLESSED TO HAVE THESE PEOPLE IN MY LIFE

5 REASONS TO BE THANKFUL

1.
2.
3.
4.
5.

NOTES:

Me Time

Write down the things that make you happy. Then, check the box every day that you spend time with that activity.

	☐ ☐ ☐ ☐ ☐ ☐ ☐
	☐ ☐ ☐ ☐ ☐ ☐ ☐
	☐ ☐ ☐ ☐ ☐ ☐ ☐
	☐ ☐ ☐ ☐ ☐ ☐ ☐
	☐ ☐ ☐ ☐ ☐ ☐ ☐
	☐ ☐ ☐ ☐ ☐ ☐ ☐
	☐ ☐ ☐ ☐ ☐ ☐ ☐
	☐ ☐ ☐ ☐ ☐ ☐ ☐

NOTES:

Self Care

DAILY INSPIRATION

WATER INTAKE:

FITNESS GOALS

One day at a time...

THANKFUL FOR

DAILY MEALS

BREAKFAST:

LUNCH:

DINNER:

SNACKS:

Personal Goals

MY SELF GOALS FOR THIS YEAR:

2 THINGS I CAN CHANGE TO MEET MY GOALS:

MY GREATEST OBSTACLE GOING FORWARD:

Good things take time

Mental Health Monitor

DAILY

_____
_____
_____
_____
_____
_____
_____
_____
_____
_____
_____
_____

WEEKLY

_____
_____
_____
_____
_____
_____
_____
_____
_____
_____
_____
_____

PERSONAL REFLECTIONS

Self Care Goals

TIME FRAME	MY GOALS	STEPS I'LL TAKE

be wild ~ be true ~ be happy

Self Care Techniques

MIND

_____
_____
_____
_____
_____
_____
_____
_____
_____
_____
_____
_____

BODY

_____
_____
_____
_____
_____
_____
_____
_____
_____
_____
_____
_____

PERSONAL REFLECTIONS

One Day at a Time

NOVEMBER

S	M	T	W	T	F	S
					1	2
3	4	5	6	7	8	9
10	11	12	13	14	15	16
17	18	19	20	21	22	23
24	25	26	27	28	29	30

NOTES & REMINDERS

Positive Thinking

SELF CARE TO DO LIST:

- [ ] _____
- [ ] _____
- [ ] _____
- [ ] _____
- [ ] _____
- [ ] _____
- [ ] _____
- [ ] _____
- [ ] _____
- [ ] _____
- [ ] _____
- [ ] _____
- [ ] _____
- [ ] _____

PHYSICAL NEEDS

EMOTIONAL NEEDS

HOW I FEEL TODAY

I WANT TO WORK ON...

Self Care Checklist

GOALS	M	T	W	T	F	S	S
Got enough rest	○	○	○	○	○	○	○
Spent time outdoors	○	○	○	○	○	○	○
Drank enough water	○	○	○	○	○	○	○
Spent time doing Something that makes me happy.	○	○	○	○	○	○	○
Went for a walk or exercised.	○	○	○	○	○	○	○
Spent time with family	○	○	○	○	○	○	○
Meditated	○	○	○	○	○	○	○
Connected with friends	○	○	○	○	○	○	○
_____	○	○	○	○	○	○	○
_____	○	○	○	○	○	○	○
_____	○	○	○	○	○	○	○

NOTES:

Mood Meter

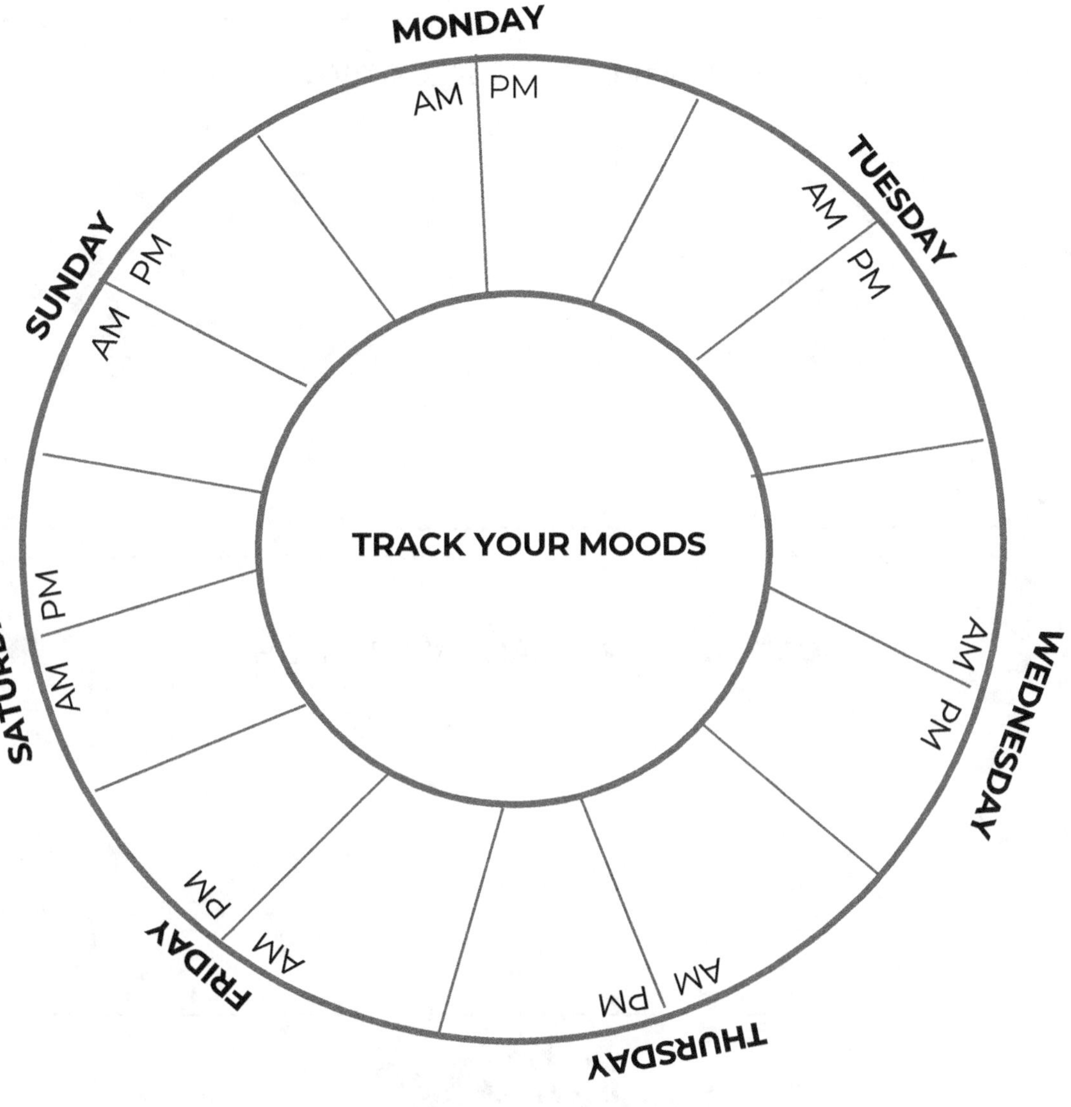
MONDAY
AM
PM
TUESDAY
AM
PM
WEDNESDAY
AM
PM
THURSDAY
AM
PM
FRIDAY
AM
PM
SATURDAY
AM
PM
SUNDAY
AM
PM
TRACK YOUR MOODS

COLOR SCALE

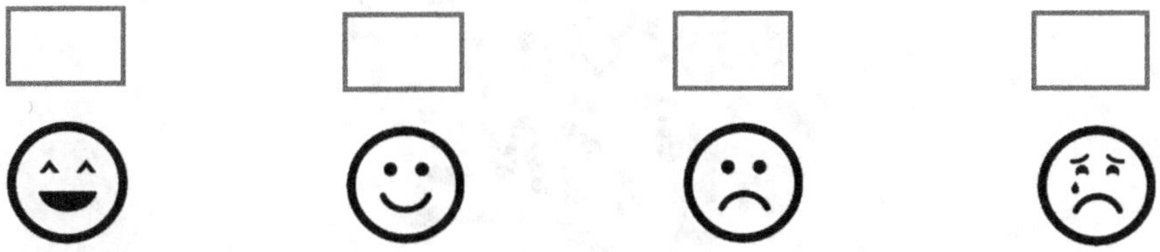

Self Care Log

HOW I CAN **MINIMIZE THE NEGATIVITY** IN MY LIFE

POSITIVE STEPS I CAN TAKE TO BE HAPPY

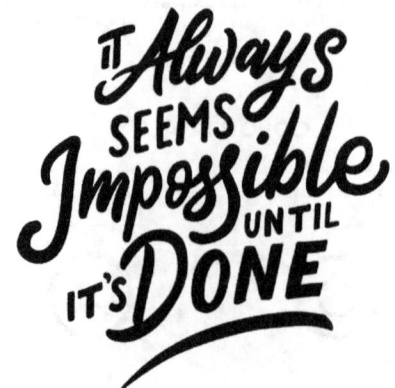

Me Time

Write down the things that make you happy. Then, check the box every day that you spend time with that activity.

NOTES:

Self Care

DAILY INSPIRATION

WATER INTAKE:

FITNESS GOALS

One day at a time...

THANKFUL FOR

DAILY MEALS

BREAKFAST:

LUNCH:

DINNER:

SNACKS:

Personal Goals

MY SELF GOALS FOR THIS YEAR:

2 THINGS I CAN CHANGE TO MEET MY GOALS:

MY GREATEST OBSTACLE GOING FORWARD:

Good things take time

Mental Health Monitor

DAILY

_____
_____
_____
_____
_____
_____
_____
_____
_____
_____
_____
_____

WEEKLY

_____
_____
_____
_____
_____
_____
_____
_____
_____
_____
_____
_____

PERSONAL REFLECTIONS

Self Care Goals

TIME FRAME	MY GOALS	STEPS I'LL TAKE

be wild ~ be true ~ be happy

Self Care Techniques

MIND

_____
_____
_____
_____
_____
_____
_____
_____
_____
_____
_____

BODY

_____
_____
_____
_____
_____
_____
_____
_____
_____
_____
_____

PERSONAL REFLECTIONS

One Day at a Time

DECEMBER

S	M	T	W	T	F	S
1	2	3	4	5	6	7
8	9	10	11	12	13	14
15	16	17	18	19	20	21
22	23	24	25	26	27	28
29	30	31				

NOTES & REMINDERS

Positive Thinking

SELF CARE TO DO LIST:

- [ ] _____
- [ ] _____
- [ ] _____
- [ ] _____
- [ ] _____
- [ ] _____
- [ ] _____
- [ ] _____
- [ ] _____
- [ ] _____
- [ ] _____
- [ ] _____
- [ ] _____
- [ ] _____

PHYSICAL NEEDS

EMOTIONAL NEEDS

HOW I FEEL TODAY

I WANT TO WORK ON...

Self Care Checklist

GOALS M T W T F S S

Got enough rest ○ ○ ○ ○ ○ ○ ○

Spent time outdoors ○ ○ ○ ○ ○ ○ ○

Drank enough water ○ ○ ○ ○ ○ ○ ○

Spent time doing Something that makes me happy. ○ ○ ○ ○ ○ ○ ○

Went for a walk or exercised. ○ ○ ○ ○ ○ ○ ○

Spent time with family ○ ○ ○ ○ ○ ○ ○

Meditated ○ ○ ○ ○ ○ ○ ○

Connected with friends ○ ○ ○ ○ ○ ○ ○

_____ ○ ○ ○ ○ ○ ○ ○

_____ ○ ○ ○ ○ ○ ○ ○

_____ ○ ○ ○ ○ ○ ○ ○

NOTES:

Mood Meter

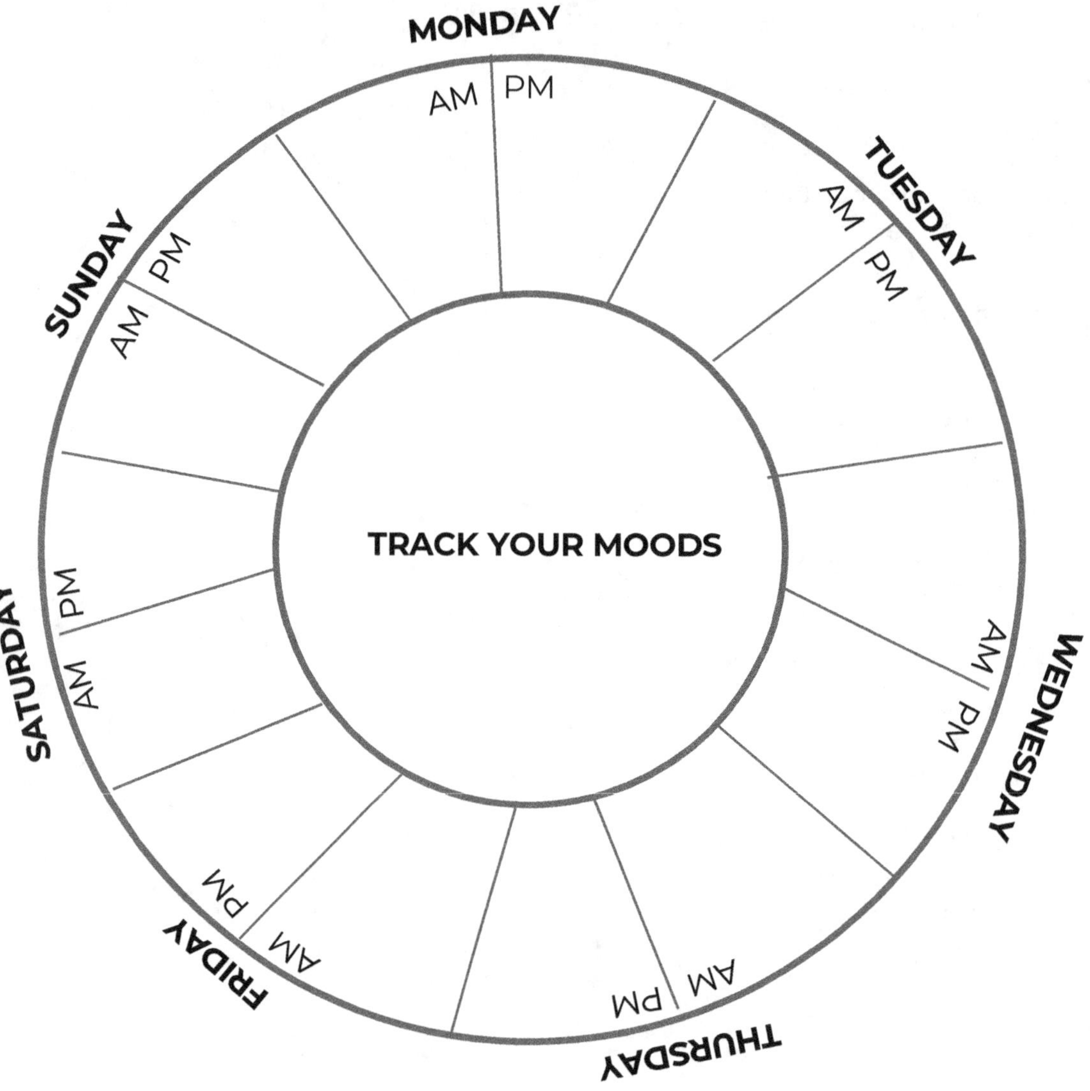
MONDAY
AM
PM
TUESDAY
AM
PM
WEDNESDAY
AM
PM
THURSDAY
AM
PM
FRIDAY
AM
PM
SATURDAY
AM
PM
SUNDAY
AM
PM
TRACK YOUR MOODS

COLOR SCALE

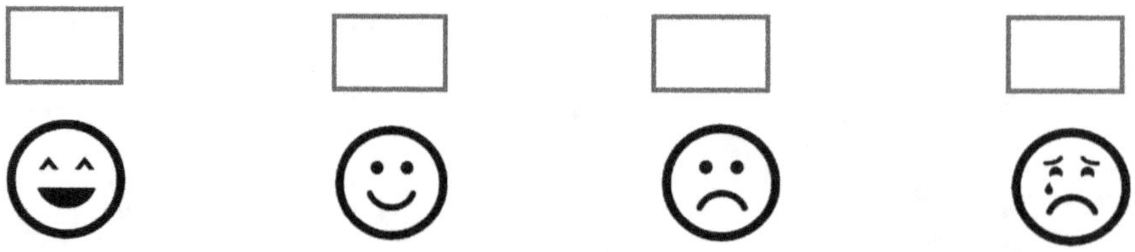

Me Time

Write down the things that make you happy. Then, check the box every day that you spend time with that activity.

Activity	M	T	W	T	F	S	S
	☐	☐	☐	☐	☐	☐	☐
	☐	☐	☐	☐	☐	☐	☐
	☐	☐	☐	☐	☐	☐	☐
	☐	☐	☐	☐	☐	☐	☐
	☐	☐	☐	☐	☐	☐	☐
	☐	☐	☐	☐	☐	☐	☐
	☐	☐	☐	☐	☐	☐	☐
	☐	☐	☐	☐	☐	☐	☐

NOTES:

Self Care

DAILY **INSPIRATION**

DAILY **MEALS**

BREAKFAST:

_____
_____
_____

LUNCH:

_____
_____
_____

DINNER:

_____
_____
_____

WATER INTAKE:

▯ ▯ ▯ ▯ ▯ ▯ ▯ ▯

FITNESS **GOALS**

_____
_____
_____

SNACKS:

_____
_____
_____
_____

One day at a time...

THANKFUL **FOR**

Personal Goals

MY SELF GOALS FOR THIS YEAR:

2 THINGS I CAN CHANGE TO MEET MY GOALS:

MY GREATEST OBSTACLE GOING FORWARD:

Good things take time

Mental Health Monitor

DAILY

WEEKLY

PERSONAL REFLECTIONS

www.ingramcontent.com/pod-product-compliance
Lightning Source LLC
Chambersburg PA
CBHW081000170526
45158CB00010B/2859